Medicare:

2018-2020:

THE COMPLETE

COMPREHENSIVE GUIDE

Mario Robertson

© 2018

Additionally, the information in the following pages is intended only for informational purposes and should thus be thought of as universal. As befitting its nature, it is presented without assurance regarding its prolonged validity or interim quality. Trademarks that are mentioned are done without written consent and can in no way be considered an endorsement from the trademark holder.

INTRODUCTION

Medicare is a government program that affects many different fields and areas: financial, medical, political, insurance, and retirement fields. It is estimated that over 55 million people received Medicare benefits in 2015, and that number continues to rise each year.

One of the reasons that Medicare is such an intricate plan is that it covers those who are either disabled or over 65 years old. Many people rely on it to get costly medical services that they would not be able to afford otherwise. With over 15% of the US population relying on Medicare, any change to it can cause confusion and concern. This is not helped by the fact that people include speculation and opinions when discussing what's available under the program.

Fortunately, there are a number of reliable sources to help you figure out what you qualify for, how to enroll in the program, and what is covered. Since there is a lot of misinformation as well (it is the Internet after all), this guide will help you through all of the basics. You will also get links and information for reliable sources so you can start getting more detailed information about your specific situation.

It is important to know that Medicare alone is not enough, it was never designed to be your only health insurance plan. Medi gap plans and supplemental insurance can ensure that you do not dip into your retirement savings to take care of unexpected medical costs. You should take the time to review your options to determine the best solution for your specific circumstances.

TABLE OF CONTENTS

CHAPTER 1. WHAT IS MEDICARE?

Medicare is often in the news because it has far reaching effects for many Americans over 65 years old (and a number of disabled Americans). For senior citizens with health issues, regular medical needs, or who are very conscious of their health care, Medicare is an essential part of their budget. It does not cover everything, but it can substantially reduce medical costs, including prescriptions.

BRIEF HISTORY

The initial idea of a nationwide insurance system for all Americans actually goes back to over 100 years ago when Theodore Roosevelt sought a third presidential term in 1912. His initial idea didn't gain any real traction for over 50 years. President Harry S. Truman was still early in his first term when he decided to call on Congress to finally create a national insurance system for the people of the United States. His idea was to cover all Americans, and not just one particular group. However, Congress was unwilling to do any real work on national health insurance for another twenty years when President John F. Kennedy started trying to push for a system to cover seniors. This push was the result of a study that indicated that over half of the senior population in the US (people over 65 years old) did not have health insurance. This created an unsustainable financial crisis for many and that was having negative effects for overall medical costs. Despite this, Congress did little to help assist seniors.

In 1965, President Lyndon B. Johnson was finally presented with legislation that would begin to help seniors with medical expenses. It was not the ideal coverage dreamed of by

Theodore Roosevelt that would have benefited all Americans, but it was at least helping one of the more vulnerable groups within the country.

The first major change to Medicare occurred in 1972 when President Richard M. Nixon signed a new piece of legislation to expand coverage to people under 65 years old who were disabled. With the Omnibus Reconciliation Act of 1980, Congress expanded the services to include various home health services. This act also saw the creation of Medigap oversight by the federal government.

For the most part, Medicare has expanded since it was signed into law in 1965. There is current political pressure to make health care coverage accessible to all Americans, not just two particular groups (senior citizens and those with long-term disabilities). Though it has changed over the years, with an increasing number of Baby Boomers becoming dependent on it, it is becoming difficult for Medicare to be altered in any way that will reduce what seniors have access to in terms of medical care and prescription medications. It now takes up about 15% of the federal budget and will likely continue to increase over the coming years as people live longer.

The Importance of Medicare

Prior to Medicare's final passage in 1965, senior citizens were facing gradually increasing costs for regular medical care. As they increasingly needed more appointments, screenings, and tests, the costs were steadily becoming too high for the small income that most seniors received through Social Security.

With life expectancy also steadily increasing, this meant that more people were finding it difficult to meet their basic needs because their medical expenses were too high. Medicare offered a solution to a growing problem among senior citizens, but it did not affect just seniors. With a growing demographic of people who were unable to meet their medical payments, the medical field was beginning to see a rise in uncollected and uncollectable debt. This meant raising costs for everyone who used medical services and products. In turn this increased the payments for additional doctor and hospital visits. It was a vicious cycle that was financially crippling an entire generation and having serious negative effects on the medical industry.

Medicare was not the perfect solution, but it did significantly alleviate the problems for the growing number of people living beyond 65 years old. It also allowed the medical profession to keep rates affordable for seniors and others who sought its help.

CHAPTER 2. COVERAGE

OVERVIEW

Within the Medicare Parts, you need to understand exactly what Medicare will cover. The next section breaks down the parts of original Medicare, and what they cover.

Your first choice will be to enroll in Parts A and B of Medicare. You can do so over the phone at (1-800-633-4227 or 1-800- MEDICARE). You may also enroll at

www.socialsecurity.gov/medicare/

Note: *"You need to be enrolled in part A and B before purchasing any additional coverage"*

THE FOUR PARTS

Medicare is divided into four parts (A, B, C, and D), each with its own specific purpose.

MEDICARE PART A

Medicare Part A is the first section of original Medicare we will cover. Part A covers all hospital visits and follow up services:

- Inpatient hospital visits and care

- Inpatient hospital visits requiring additional time, and it covers the majority of facilities with skilled nurses

- Home health services and hospice care

Though Part A is part of the original plan, not every service currently covered was included in the original plan. For related expenses approved by Congress, updates for hospital visits, and required care after leaving a hospital are added to this part.

Deductible: Part A of Medicare has a $1,340 deductible, which the insured would responsible to pay each benefit period, "every 60 days." Remember the insured pays the deductible before the coverage picks up the difference.

Example: You receive a bill for $5,000 from the hospital, you pay the first $1,340, and Medicare pays the difference.

MEDICARE PART B

Medicare Part B is the other half of the original Medicare plan. It is intended to cover the majority of regular medical coverage that is not associated with inpatient hospital costs. This does include some services that may be used during a hospital visit, but these are services that could be provided outside of the hospital as well.

- Visits to doctors and for results for clinical lab services

- Outpatient hospital costs and preventative medical costs

- The majority of surgical fees, surgical supplies, and screenings

- Occupational and physical therapy

- Home health care

- Durable Medical Equipment

Because it covers preventative costs, Part B applies to any shots that are part of that care, such as annual flu shots.

Part B of Medicare for most Americans will cost around $134 per month.

Part B of Original Medicare also has a annual deductible of $183, in addition the insured is responsible for 20% coinsurance of the bill.

Example: You have a $100,000-dollar bill for a treatment covered under part B, you the insured would pay the deductible of $183 plus the 20% coinsurance of the bill for $20,000, and Medicare pays the difference.

Authors note: As you can see original Medicare can leave you exposed to high deductibles and copays, we will now look at two different options that can cover the gaps from Original Medicare, these will be explained as (1) Medicare advantage plans, and (2) Medigap plans, also known as "Supplemental plans."

MEDICARE PART C

Medicare Part C is simply the combination of both Part A and Part B along with additional coverage offered through a private insurer. Most Medicare advantage plans include Part D "Prescription Drug Plan," (covered in the next section), making it easier to track all costs associated with medical needs. There are four plans available under Part C

- HMO or HMO-POS plans (Health Maintenance Organizations)

- PPO plans (Preferred Provider Organizations)

- PFFS plans (Private Fee-for Service)

- SNP plans (Special Needs Plans)

The primary difference between Part C and the other parts is that it must be obtained through a private health care insurance provider. This is done under insurance companies Medicare Advantage plans. It means paying less out of pocket as well, and can include other medical perks, such as vision, basic dental, and hearing screenings.

Authors Note: Medicare Advantage plans are always better than just having traditional Medicare, as they don't leave you exposed to extreme copays that are uncapped. With most plans, once you have reached your Maximum Out of Pocket amount, (Varies Per Plan) your out of pocket medical expenses stop for the remainder of the year. Medicare advantage plans do not cover as much as supplemental plans, however if you are on a budget they are the best bet.

Medicare Advantage plans also change based on your geographic location, you will find less plans offered in rural areas, and many plans offered in populated and retirement areas, (Florida) A Medicare advantage plan can be as low as $0 per month or higher, the price in this case is irrelevant, as a $0 premium plan could be better than a $40 plan, it is simply a matter of what is available in your area geographically.

WHY DOES IT MATTER WHERE I LIVE FOR MEDICARE ADVANTAGE PLANS?

Remember these plans are offered through private insurers, so they are allowed to choose which states they want to create a presence to be competitive in. Humana for example may cover an area AARP does not. You will need to do a little research if you are interested in

MAPD's (Medicare Advantage Plans) to see which plan suits your needs the best.

HMO vs PPO:

HMO plans mean you need to stay within your plans network in order to be covered. Both your doctor and hospital must be in network with the HMO in order to qualify for coverage. "Emergencies are the exception." HMO plans typically are the most cost effective MAPD.

HMO plans also require a PCP (Primary Care Physician) to be referred to a specialist.

PPO plans: mean it is cheaper for you to utilize doctors and hospitals in network, however you may be visit doctors and hospitals out of the network, but you will typically pay a higher copay.

(Please Note, Chapter 4 covers Medigap plans which are the most comprehensive plans in Medicare, and my personal recommendation for all Medicare recipients who can afford it.)

MEDICARE PART D

Medicare Part D was created to cover prescription costs, making it easier to track the costs of prescription medications for seniors and those with long-term disabilities. It also provides a way to obtain Medicare without the other parts. You can get Part D as a stand-alone plan or as part of other medical coverage (such as a Medicare Advantage Plan). Part D has only one purpose and that is to help cover the cost of prescriptions.

Part D is the only part that is used in conjunction with the other three parts. It is necessary to present your card for Part D when you purchase your prescriptions.

You will need to check your eligibility (Chapter 3) to determine which parts you can use.

THE IMPORTANCE OF THE MEDICARE PARTS

Ultimately, the Medicare Part or Parts that you choose will determine the kind of coverage you have. There are more options under Part C, but it also requires going through a private provider, which is not an option available to everyone. Check out Chapter 3 to get a better understanding of the different eligibility requirements to get a better idea of what your coverage is.

For many, the **cost** is the biggest determiner of which Medicare Part to select.

NEW PARTICIPANTS

Coverage for new participants is largely the same as for existing participants. The primary difference in coverage is related to the

Medicare Part or Parts in which you enroll. The biggest difference is that you will need to meet the waiting period before your Medicare coverage will begin. Instead of having coverage that carries over, you will need to wait for the first day of the month after your application is received and approved.

The majority of questions related to Medicare focus on Part D since that is the area where most people require the most help. Chapter 5 covers details you need to know about prescriptions covered under Medicare. The best way to determine if something is covered is to contact your provider and ask about specific coverage. If you require Part A, it is best to go ahead and get Part B (and vice versa) because you want to ensure that you have adequate coverage for both regular care and emergency medical costs.

Note that it is illegal for any insurance company in the Health Insurance Marketplace to try to sell you other insurance if they know that you are on Medicare. Be cautious if you need to contact the Marketplace and let them know that you are on or are applying for Medicare. If you have not been accepted yet, they may be able to offer you a plan in case you do not qualify, but they cannot contact you about plans once you are an active Medicare participant.

Also, many clinical trials can be covered by Medicare. If there are other medical costs, a definitive diagnosis as a result of the trial, or complications from the trial, these will also be covered by Medicare. Make sure to ask about any associated costs, tools, and items that may be required by the trial so that you can verify its coverage before you commit to the trial. Some types of trials may have associated costs that are not covered either because they do not qualify or because they are experimental.

EXISTING PARTICIPANTS

The majority of the coverage that you currently have under Medicare will remain the same in the coming year. Check out Chapter 6 for anticipated changes based on the current rules and laws passed regarding Medicare.

Chapter 3. Enrollment and

Eligibility

Besides the types of coverage offered under Medicare, the greatest changes to the program has been in eligibility and enrollment periods.

The Annual Enrollment period for 2018 is from October 15th to December 7th.

Authors Note:

(Please note the annual enrollment period only pertains to Medicare Advantage Plans (MAPD) and Part D plans, supplemental plans can be applied for anytime of the year, however you may be required to go through the underwriting process.)

If you are aging into Medicare (age 65) you have 3 months before you turn 65, and 3 months after you turn 65 to qualify for guaranteed enrollment in either a MAPD or Supplemental plan. There are some carriers which will allow you to enroll as early as 6 months in advance of turning 65 for Medigap Plans. **This means you cannot be turned down for pre-existing conditions.** The only condition MAPD's will turn you down for is ESRD (End Stage Renal Disease), however supplemental plans are much stricter, so be sure and **take advantage of your guaranteed enrollment opportunity.**

What if I'm still employed past the age of 65 using company insurance and have not signed up for Medicare?

You still qualify for guaranteed issue, you should be in touch with an insurance agent at least 3 months prior to leaving your employee insurance to ensure a smooth transition into Medicare.

This does not give you much time to look at your options, something that this book can help you to better understand (reducing the number of questions you will have for the insurance agent). It will also make it easier to pinpoint the questions you need to ask should you have any about your specific situation. Check out Appendix A for links if you have other questions about enrollment or your eligibility.

ANNUAL ENROLLMENT PERIOD

The enrollment period is for both new and existing Medicare participants. For those who are newly eligible, you have the chance to choose which Medicare Part is best for you, or if you would like to combine several parts for a more comprehensive medical plan. Note that you do need Part B to meet current federal requirements for insurance coverage – Part A alone does not meet federal regulations for insurance coverage.

The following are the types of decisions you will need to make during the enrollment period.

• You can change from Parts A and B to Part C, (Which simply means to purchase a Medicare advantage plan because it combines part A, B, and usually part D)

• If you have found a preferable Medicare Advantage plan, you can switch to it during this time. The same is true for your Medicare Part D plan.

• You can enroll in Part D by itself or add it if you do not currently have it with your other Medicare parts. Note that there could be an applicable late enrollment penalty if you have been enrolled in other parts and excluded Part D up to this point.

For those already enrolled in Medicare, you may not need to do anything during the enrollment period. This period is really for people who wish to make changes to their current plan. For those who are already enrolled in a Medicare Advantage Plan, you will need to verify that your plan is not changing or being discontinued. If the plan is changing or being discontinued, you will need to sign up saying that you want to enroll in the updated plan. If your plan is being discontinued, you need to find a new plan for next year. You should receive a notice that your plan is being discontinued, but taking the initiative to verify it now will give you more time to start looking into other plans. If you have moved since last year, it also ensures that you know to look for other coverage in case the letter does not reach you.

Even if your plan does not change, your premium may increase, so you need to at least verify your premium for 2018. Checking your premium may result in a decision to change plans. You also should make sure that the coverage you have still meets your needs. If you have been diagnosed with any medical conditions, have had a change in medication, or rely on certain aspects of your current coverage, you need to check coverage for next year to ensure that you have what you need going forward. It is possible that a quick check will result in you finding a different plan that more closely meets your needs. Even if you plan to allow your coverage to auto-renew, make sure that it is the plan you need before the enrollment period closes.

DISENROLLMENT PERIOD

If you enrolled in a Medicare Advantage Plan but decide that it is not right for you, the period between January 1 and February 14 is the disenrollment period specifically for switching back to original Medicare Parts A and B. Notice that you cannot switch to another Medicare Advantage plan during this time, and you cannot change from Parts A and B to a Medicare Advantage Plan.

It is possible to switch Medicare Advantage plans outside of either enrollment period if you qualify for a Special Enrollment Period. The next section covers who is eligible during this period.

You can also enroll in Medicare Part D plan during this time if you leave a Medicare Advantage plan. Your Part D plan will become effective the first day of the month after the month in which you enroll. For example, if you enroll on January 15, your Part D coverage will begin February 1. If you enroll in Part D on February 10, your coverage will begin on March 1.

GENERAL ENROLLMENT PERIOD

If you did not enroll for Medicare A or B during your Initial Enrollment Period (3-1-3) you will be given another opportunity to do so between January 1 to March 31 of each year. This is called the General Enrollment Period (GEP) Note that your coverage will not be effective until July 1 – but you will then have both Medicare parts. This does mean that you could be subject to a late enrollment fee for not having adequate coverage for part of the year. Your penalty will vary based on how many months over a 12 month period you were uninsured even though you were eligible.

ELIGIBILITY

Most people over 65 years old are eligible for Medicare, but they are no longer the only group who can participate in Medicare plans. Those with qualifying long-term disabilities are also eligible. The following are some guidelines to help you determine your eligibility.

• Anyone who is retired and receiving benefits through either Social Security or the Railroad Retirement Board can look into the different Medicare options.

• Anyone who is eligible for either Social Security or Railroad Retirement Board but hasn't yet finished filing for those benefits can also begin enrolling in Medicare.

- Government employees and their spouses who are eligible through a Medicare-covered agency.

To be eligible for a premium-free Part A plan, you must meet both of the following criteria.

- You must be over 65 years of age.

- You or your spouse must have paid taxes to Medicare for a minimum of 10 years.

If you do not meet these requirements, you may still be eligible for Part A coverage, but you will need to pay a premium.

Those with a qualifying disability must meet slightly different requirements. Whether you are eligible for a premium-free Part A plan can vary based on the severity of the disability and how long you have paid taxes or how long you have qualified for Social Security or Railroad Retirement Board disability benefits.

To determine if you are eligible for Medicare coverage, you can go to Medicare.gov eligibility to check. There is also a calculator to help you determine what your premium will be for Parts A and B. The calculator does include other possible options, but it is not comprehensive. If you have further questions, you can contact someone at the Medicare service desk for details.

MEDICARE ADVANTAGE PLAN

ELIGIBILITY

The rules for eligibility are different for Part C than the other parts. You must meet the following three criteria to be eligible to enroll in a Medicare Advantage Plan.

• You need to currently be enrolled in both Medicare Parts A and B.

• You must be a resident within the service area of the plan in which you wish to enroll.

• You cannot have been diagnosed as having End-Stage Renal Disease. There are some other exceptions, so you may want to verify if you can enroll by contacting one of the resources listed in Appendix A.

SPECIAL ENROLLMENT PERIOD

For those who were still working during their Initial Enrollment period (turning 65) and missed this period because you were covered by an employer's health care plan can qualify during this period. From the time your job ends or if you lose creditable coverage from your employer, you have eight-months to enroll into Part B, and this period starts the month following the end of your job or the month your other health care coverage ends – whichever time occurs first. You then have 60 days to enroll into a Medicare Advantage Plan (MAPD) or choose a Medigap Plan. Please note that this time frame does not allow you to enroll into a Part D plan unless you choose to enroll into a MAPD and it includes Part D coverage.

CHAPTER 4. MEDIGAP PLANS

(MEDICARE SUPPLEMENT)

Most Medicare plans are not free, so you do need to know how much it will cost per month to have Medicare coverage. The cost largely depends on which part or parts best meet your needs.

Medicare is a great safety net for those who qualify, but it may not cover all of the medical costs you incur after you qualify. Since you never know when you will experience health problems, there is the risk that your medical costs could exceed your financial capabilities (especially if you are retired). The best way to ensure that you don't have to go back to work or suffer severe financial hardships because of unexpected medical costs is to have supplemental coverage, also known as Medigap coverage. These plans will increase your regular healthcare costs due to premiums, but in the event that something goes wrong, you will have the insurance you need to keep you from more severe financial stress at a time when you don't need any additional anxiety. Taking advantage of the additional medical coverage when you are eligible can be a literal life saver, particularly if you have a pre-existing condition. Your approval is guaranteed, but many people are not aware that it is an option.

This chapter covers costs and the period when you will be able to get Medigap coverage.

MEDICARE COST OVERVIEW

Medicare is covered in large part by taxpayers, but there are costs that you will need to pay. If you have Medicare Part C, you will have an agreement with your provider for your monthly premium costs. For those on Medicare Part B, the average premium cost for 2017 is $134 a month. This average does vary based on individual income, but it is a good baseline for those who are researching costs. If you are eligible for Social Security benefits as well, the premium is more likely to be around $110 a month. In most cases, there is not a premium cost for Part A. it is possible to purchase Part A if it isn't already free, but the costs are considerably higher (between $200 and $420).

You will be expected to pay some fees for visits to hospitals and doctors. This is similar to a copay, which begins after you have met your deductible. Currently the deductible is under $200 ($183). Once the deductible is met, you will pay 20% for all approved costs.

MEDIGAP PLANS

Medicare can help those who qualify for it, but it doesn't necessarily cover everything you may need. Whether you are healthy or not, Medigap plans are something everyone should consider once they are eligible for Medicare. All new Medicare enrollees are guaranteed to be approved for a Medigap plan, although you will probably choose a plan based on the cost of your plan, which vary considerably. .

Before seeing a doctor, you will need to ask if the practice participates in Medicare. As long as your doctor is a participant, your Medigap Plan is required to make payments to your doctor at your request in the event that Medicare does not cover the complete cost.

THE MEDIGAP BASICS

Remember you have 6 months (90 days with some carriers) before aging into Medicare, and 5 months after aging in, to qualify for Open Enrollment. In this period, you cannot be turned down for Pre-Existing conditions.

Medigap is a type of supplemental insurance for people who are eligible for Medicare. It is sold by private insurance companies and acts as a secondary insurance when Medicare does not cover all of a person's medical costs. It can be used to pay for things like copayments and deductibles, as well as being an insurance you may be able to use if you travel abroad. Medicare cannot cover you if you decide to travel after retirement, but some Medigap plans can. Your Medigap Policy does not begin to pay for medical costs until Medicare has covered all amounts that are approved for coverage. Essentially, you use Medigap to cover your medical costs once your available Medicare budget is used, or if you travel abroad (if your plan covers travel abroad).

States can provide as many as 10 Medigap plans for their enrollees however I will focus on the top 2.

MEDIGAP PLAN F

This is the most comprehensive plan available as it covers 100% of the cost Medicare does not. So long as you pay the monthly premium for this plan, you will not receive any other bills. 100% of doctor and hospital bills are covered. The one thing not covered under any supplemental plan is Part D, Prescription drug plan, which is purchased separate from the Medigap plans.

(Please note Plan F will no longer be available after 2020, however if you enroll before the deadline, you may keep the plan indefinitely)

MEDIGAP PLAN G

This plan is the exact same as Plan F except it has an annual deductible of $183 "Yes this is from your part B of Medicare, this is not a separate deductible." This plan is typically cheaper than Plan F, and usually the best value for your money.

Authors Note: Medigap plans are accepted by any doctor or hospital that accepts Medicare, by law, they must accept your Medigap plan. In addition you can clearly see how comprehensive Medigap plans are in comparison to Medicare Advantage plans. Pay the monthly premium, and avoid hospital and doctor bills all together!

There are more plans offered than F and G, however they offer less coverage. You would need to inquire with your insurance agent for specifications.

Lastly many Medigap plans offer international coverage, verify the amount with your agent.

The benefits must meet a set standard, regardless of the state offering the plan. In other words, Plan F and G as well as the other Medigap Plans not mentioned are the exact same plan no matter where you purchase it. Massachusetts, Minnesota, and Wisconsin are the three exceptions to this. They have their own set of standardized benefits, typically providing better benefits for their participants.

Though they are regulated by the federal government, Medigap plans are offered by private insurers, and that means the prices are going to vary, possibly substantially. If you are looking at three different Medigap Plan F policies offered by three different companies, you may be looking at three very different premiums, even though the plans are the exact same, and required to be by law. Keep in mind that price is not necessarily an indication that a plan is better or worse. The more important aspect to pay attention to here would be, is the company you are purchasing insurance from, an A+ rated company through the Better business Bureau? Also, the companies that sell Medigap plans must be licensed to do so. Make sure to verify a company's coverage before committing to paying a premium.

Finally, Medigap does not cover prescription medications. The only way to cover prescription costs is to have Medicare Part D. That does mean that you will have three multiple different medical plans to juggle, but considering how expensive health care can be upon retirement age, it is probably worth the investment of time to make sure you have all of the bases covered.

MEDIGAP ELIGIBILITY

As soon as you qualify to receive Medicare, you are also eligible for Medigap coverage. You do have a limited amount of time to enroll in Medigap plans, so you need to make sure to get started as early as possible. Most people miss the opportunity for additional insurance because they do not realize that they qualify for more coverage. Since the time frame for enrolling for Medigap coverage is limited, you do need to make sure to do your research before your eligibility period expires.

In addition to enrolling during the eligibility time frame, you have to have both Medicare Part A and B to apply for Medigap. That does mean you will need to pay the Medicare Part B premium in addition to the Medigap premium every month. Also, it cannot cover more than a single person. Medicare plans are always individual plans, not family plans. You and your spouse if applicable will each have your own Medicare number and policy number.

Once you have the Medigap plan, you are guaranteed to be able to renew it, regardless of any health issues you develop once the coverage starts. As long as you pay your premium every month, your insurance company cannot cancel your plan.

You cannot have both Medigap coverage and Medicare Advantage Plan, nor can you have Medigap and a Medicare Medical Savings Account Plan. Medigap provides coverage for those who can afford an additional policy. It covers more than both Medicare Advantage Plan and Medicare Medical Savings Accounts, so if you can afford the additional monthly premium, it can actually save you a lot of money if you have a medical emergency or need additional care.

Though it does cover more than most of the other types of Medicare plans, Medigap does not cover all of your medical needs. You will need separate coverage for vision and dental. It does not cover items like regular medical devices and tools, such as glasses and hearing aids. It also will not cover long-term care or a private nurse.

MEDIGAP COST

For most people Medigap is the best solution to ensuring that they have more comprehensive healthcare coverage. However, it does come with a cost that will increase at a rate of about 3-5% annually. The cost does vary by company, state, and plan, which can make finding the right solution for you a more time-consuming endeavor than you may initially expect.

The price for a Medigap Plan is usually based on three factors.

• **Community-rated** plans are based on the area that you live in, not your age. The price will go up based on factors like inflation.

• **Issue-age rated** plans have a cost that is based on your age group. If you join at the youngest eligible age range, you will have a cheaper cost than those who join at a later age. Your rate will go up based on inflation and economic factors, but not your age.

• **Attained-age rated** plans are based on your age when you join, and then the price goes up as you age. This means that you can pay less than others when you join, but your costs will go up over time based on your age and inflation, so you could end up paying considerably more in premiums in 10 years' time.

Like other insurance plans, they do take other factors into account when setting your premium, such as if you are a non-smoker.

CHANGING OR DROPPING A MEDIGAP PLAN

Given the three primary types of plans and costs, you may decide to switch plans later. You do need to be careful because you may get charged additional fees for making the change at the wrong time. Most of the fees stem from policies that were in effect before 2006 when prescription drugs could be included. For those who want to switch to a policy that does not include prescription drugs, visit the Medicare site for details on fees and changing to a new plan that does not include prescriptions. You can also contact Customer Service if you have any questions.

WHY IT HELPS

When you first qualify for Medicare, there is a good chance that it will be enough, at least for a little while. The problem is that by the time you qualify for it, you have a greater chance of unexpected healthcare needs. Even if you don't have a major health event, the costs of staying healthy will increase regularly. You will need a new prescription for blood pressure medication or more frequent visits to your doctor for regular pains. Even your regular health care preventative costs are going to increase because you are going to need to go to the doctor more often for more tests. It is just a part of aging – you will go to the doctor more and you are more likely to need more medication or monitoring. Medicare is great, but it doesn't cover everything. Medigap provides you with a way of offsetting medical emergencies and increasing medical needs over time. It is essentially an investment in your medical future. Since you never know when you are going to need more coverage, it is a good idea to get a Medigap Plan now.

MEDICARE ADVANTAGE PLANS

If you do not want a Medigap plan, or if you find that you can no longer afford the increasing premiums of your plan, you do have another option.

You cannot have both a Medicare Advantage Plan and a Medigap Plan. It is an either or situation, and typically a person's budget determines which plan a person will choose. Medicare Advantage Plans are not free, but they are less costly than most Medigap Plans. They do require that you have Medicare Parts

A and B, but the premiums are typically lower than Medigap Plans. You will need to review available plans and companies (they are offered by private companies). To help you in your research you can use the Medicare site's Medicare's Plan Finder to get started.

Most Medicare Advantage Plans are based on copayments, and those will vary by company, and they vary greatly based on the area you live in. For example, many parts of Florida have a $0 copay for your primary care physician.

It is not as comprehensive as Medigap, but it is a better choice than not having any supplemental insurance. Medical costs are almost guaranteed to go up as you age, so having additional coverage can save you a lot of financial stress. This is a good alternative for people who cannot afford Medigap or who find their Medigap premiums are becoming a financial burden.

OTHER MEDICARE SUPPLEMENTS

Medigap and Medicare Advantage Plans are the g0-to plans for Medicare recipients, but you can get other supplemental plans through private insurance companies if you need additional coverage. For government employees and people who are in unions, you may be able to get better coverage with a long-term solution through your former employer. Veterans also qualify for additional healthcare benefits. For everyone else, Medigap and Medicare Advantage Plan provide a steadier, more reliable supplement because you cannot be denied coverage if something happens. You do run that risk with other private insurance policies.

CHAPTER 5 - PRESCRIPTIONS

Prescriptions are treated differently under Medicare than under any private insurance. Medicare covers prescriptions under Part D. It can be used in addition to other types of insurance, as well as being added to your coverage with Parts A and B. There are a lot of rules and regulations related to Part D if you use it with other types of insurance or government programs (such as Medicaid which varies by state), so it is best to go directly to the Medicare website to look up the specifics.

This chapter covers the basics of Part D so that you can have an idea of what you will get when you enroll in Part D, even if it is the only part of Medicare in which you enroll. Given how many medications you are likely to need as you age, it is nearly a guarantee that you will want to enroll in Part D, even if you have other healthcare insurance.

ELIGIBILITY AND ENROLLMENT

When you first become eligible for Medicare, you need to enroll in Part D to ensure that you do not end up paying a penalty for enrolling late. There are two instances where you may not be charged a late penalty fee if you don't enroll for Part D when you first become eligible.

• You have prescription drug coverage through other means. There are some rules and restrictions on what is considered creditable coverage, so if you are not sure whether your coverage meets the requirements, contact the Medicare Customer Service to ask about your specific situation.

• You require Extra Help because of financial hardship or limited resources. Extra Help is provided for enrollees who do not have adequate financial resources to cover the costs for prescription medication.

Just like Parts A, B, and C, you will be able to review your Medicare Part D coverage annually. If you do not want to change anything, your existing plans will automatically renew. You will have the annual opportunity to review your coverage and change it in case your needs have changed. The Medicare Administration has created a short video to help you understand Medicare Parts C and D since they are not as straight forward as Parts A and B.

Every American is considered eligible when they turn 65, even if you decide to continue working.

•   You can actually start the enrollment process up to three months before you turn 65, and your Part D coverage will begin the day that you turn 65.

•   If you wait to enroll around or after your 65th birthday, your benefits will begin the first day of the month after your birthday.

•   You can wait up to three months after you turn 65 to enroll. If you do, your benefits will begin the first day of the following month after you enroll.

You must enroll by the end of the third month after your 65th birthday to enroll on time.

There are two enrollment periods.

•   You can enroll during your Initial Enrollment Period (3-1-3, turning 65) or the Annual Enrollment Period which is October 15 to December 7 of every year. (Please note that waiting to enroll to into Part D during the Annual Enrollment Period may incur a Late Enrollment Penalty (LEP)

•   If you have Medicare Advantage and you want to cancel your plan, you can do that during January to February 14 (Disenrollment Period). During this time you can also enroll in Part D to make sure you have prescription coverage.

You can enroll during some periods outside of the regular Medicare enrollment period, but you may be charged a late enrollment penalty for doing so. It may also be too late to enroll if you do not do so during one of the applicable enrollment time frames. It is only possible to enroll in Part D outside of the scheduled Medicare enrollment periods if you have a qualifying life event that changes your situation. The enrollment period starts on the date of the life change and is called a special election period.

You may also be charged a late fee for failing to enroll when you first become eligible for Medicare. This is one of the main reasons why it is best to enroll in all applicable Medicare Parts that you need as soon as you become eligible (or even shortly before your 65th birthday). Most people end up enrolling in Part D because it can be used in conjunction with nearly every other type of insurance. Since you are nearly guaranteed to need prescription medication as you age, it just makes sense to enroll so that you have coverage when you need it. It will save you time and money later, and you are already looking at related coverage with the other parts. If you need to make adjustments later you can, but people usually keep their Part D coverage once they have it.

COST AND COVERAGE

Medicare Part D is not free, so you will need to budget the regular premium into your budget.

If you have other prescription coverage, you need to read all of the relevant material on it before enrolling in Part D. It may not make sense to pay for Part D if you have better coverage through a retirement insurance plan from your employer. Contact the Medicare Administration if you aren't sure about whether you should carry multiple types of prescription coverage.

The cost for Part D is actually complicated to calculate because it can vary from person to person and is heavily dependent on several factors:

- The prescription medications you need

- Which plan you choose

- If your regular pharmacist is considered to be in the Part D network

- If the medications you need are part of the plan's formulary of covered prescriptions

- If you qualify for Extra Help.

There are four different stages that you will also need to consider in a Part D plan:

- Premium costs

- Annual deductible

- Initial Coverage

- Coverage Gap (donut hole) See more on this below

Coverage is just as complicated because it varies based on a number of factors as well. The primary factor is the list of prescriptions that are covered under your specific plan. Depending on the tier that your medication is in for the plan, the price will vary. Changes can also be made to your prescription coverage list. When you receive any communication on your Part D coverage, you need to make sure to review it because it could include changes to prescriptions you use.

- Your provider must provide written notice at a minimum of 60 days before the effective date of any change to the prescription list.

•   If you get a refill on your prescription and a change is approaching, your provider must provide written notice and a 60-day supply of the prescription that you refilled. This ensures that you have a supply of the medication you need in case there is a cost increase. This gives you two months to rework your budget around medication that you must take regularly.

COVERAGE GAP

This is a complicated and costly part of Part D. Please note that *not everyone* will enter the coverage gap often times referred to as the donut hole of Medicare. It is probably a big relief to know that the Coverage Gap is due to go away in the year 2020. Until then, it is important to understand the basics of this phase. The Coverage Gap for 2018 will begin when the retail cost of your medications (meaning what you and your Part D plan pay collectively) reaches $3,750 you hit the donut hole. You will start paying more for the costs of your medications. You will pay 44% of the cost for generic medications and 35% of the cost for brand name medications or generics treated as brand name. When the retail amount of your meds reaches $5,000 *(note that you pay the full difference in cost between the amounts of $3,750 and $5,000) you* then hit the catastrophic phase and all of your prescription costs go down in price significantly. The Coverage Gap/Donut Hole is the same for all Part D coverage whether you have a standalone Part D plan or a Medicare Advantage Plan with Part D coverage(MAPD). It is your medications which put you in the donut hole, not the plan.

MEDICARE ADVANTAGE PLAN PART

C

You can also get prescription coverage through Medicare Advantage Plan Part C. This is offered through private insurance companies, and not through the government. It is possible that you can have Medicare Part D with Part C if you choose this type of coverage and you will not need a separate Part D plan if this is the case. However, to qualify for Medicare Advantage Plan Part C, you do have to have Medicare Parts A and B. This is a requirement to join the Medicare Advantage Plan.

You may be un-enrolled from Medicare Advantage Plan Part C under a few circumstances. If you are interested in comparing this plan with Part D, contact the Medicare Administration to see which plan is the better option for your specific circumstance. This will help ensure you don't have to deal with complications and being un-enrolled from coverage you need later.

CHAPTER 6 – CHANGES IN 2018

While Medicare is something that is often discussed, the specifics are rarely addressed in the voluminous media coverage. This is in part because the changes are so complicated and varied that it is difficult to provide all of the details individuals need to know. However, every year there are changes to Medicare. The best way to ensure that you have the coverage you need is to keep an eye on the changes and to stay in the know.

The changes to 2018 are largely on the books, making it easy for you to start reviewing the information you need to be familiar with for the year. You need to dedicate several hours to reviewing your coverage and the changes which you can do by speaking with a qualified agent . This chapter does provide an overview, but it is not comprehensive, and every individual has different needs. If you are uncertain if something you need is affected, contact the Medicare Administration to get details specific to your situation.

There are numerous changes, but the following are the biggest changes to Medicare that you need to know if you are already covered under the program.

NEW CARDS

New healthcare cards are expected, but for 2018 there will be a major change – the cards will no longer include your Social Security Number. Since it is recommended that people not carry their Social Security Cards on their person, having the number on your Medicare card (which you have to carry with you everywhere) seems like a potential security issue. The Medicare Administration listened to participants and had the number removed for new cards starting in 2018.

Each card will now come with a unique Medicare Number. This will be your new identifier when you go to the doctor or the hospital. That information will need to be updated by your regular physician, but it should not change your coverage with that physician – at least not on its own. You will need to review your Medicare Plan for specific changes to the plan.

Do NOT just throw your old card away because that puts you at risk of identity theft. When you get your new card, make sure to cut up or shred your old card. Since it has your Social Security information on it, you want to make sure that it is completely destroyed to reduce the chance that someone will find it and use that number to steal your identity.

MEDICARE PART D WILL COST LESS

Another positive change for 2018 is that prescription medication premiums are likely going to decrease for you in 2018. This is in large part thanks to a number of rebates that are being issued on prescriptions. Because rebates were originally predicted to be lower than they will actually be, people who have Medicare Part D will see a decline in their costs. It is also likely that a decrease in generic drug costs is helping to reduce premium prices. If you are able to buy generic prescriptions, this means you may be able to shift your budget a bit to put the money you save elsewhere.

You should still take the time to compare your Part D plan with other plans in case you can save more money through a different type of coverage. Simply accepting the change as being adequate could mean that you pay more than necessary. If you find that Part D is still your best option, you can enjoy the lowered premiums without having to completely redo your budget.

PART B CHANGES FOR HIGHER EARNERS AND NOT AT ALL FOR OTHER PARTICIPANTS

The change in Part B is far more complicated, but largely only affects those who earn over $85,000 a year for those who are single or $170,000 for those who are married. It will mean an increase in premiums for those who have higher incomes.

For many people, Part B is not likely to see a cost increase that is out of the expected range – and in some cases they may not change at all. While those who earn a higher income could see a more substantial increase, it is possible for those who earn less to see their premiums remain the same. For new participants, this is certainly good news. For those who have been protected under the "hold harmless" clause, it could mean losing money because this clause is closely tied with Social Security, and typically the premiums are taken directly from Social Security checks. If you need more information, contact the Medicare Administration for details so that you can appropriately budget your medical expenses for the coming year.

CHANGES TO MEDICARE ADVANTAGE MAY COST YOU MORE

Medicare Advantage has been gaining in popularity since 2005, resulting in an increase in enrollment. In 2005, roughly 13% of participants opted for Medicare Advantage over Medicare, and that went up to 30% by

2015. Because participants can also get vision, hearing, and dental coverage, it seems like a much more streamlined way of getting all of the necessary coverage.

For 2018, that steady increase in enrollment is going to start hitting the pockets of those who have Medicare Advantage, and it is coming in the form of fewer options for out-of-pocket plans. The option has always varied based on where you live, but they will be less financially friendly for 2018. Participants may be able to get a monthly premium plan that is $0, but your out-of-pocket expenses are likely to be higher. If you don't have to pay for a premium every month, but you end up having to pay $500 for prescriptions until you meet your out-of-pocket deductible that is now capped at $6,000 meaning you are paying four months more for medication than you did in 2017 with a cap of $4,000. This can cause a significant strain on finances, something that you may not be able to take. That is why it is so important to take the time to compare your current plan with others. The changes every year can mean making a switch to a different Medicare Part or plan will save you money, or at least keep your healthcare expenses relatively stable.

APPENDIX A – LINKS, FORMS,

AND ASSISTANCE

There are a number of sites with information about Medicare, but they are not equal. If you have questions or would like to learn more, you can check out these sites to get more information.

MEDICARE SITES

Medicare.gov is the official government site for everything related to Medicare. It has contact information, details, forms, and everything you need to know about this essential resource. During certain times of years you may find it a bit slow and contacting the site for assistance will take longer, but it is the site where you should always begin to look for answers.

CMS.gov is a site that is part of the Centers for Medicare and Medicaid Services, and you can set it as another one of your go to sites for questions, issues, and latest news. Dedicate some time to reviewing everything they have available so that you know where to go for the information you need.

The Medicare Resources site is a great site for a more personal look at Medicare. You can find information on supplemental insurance, Medigap coverage, and other information. However, you will need to learn to navigate through a number of ads and other information because it is not run by the government.

Medicare.com is a good starting point for researching Medicare in your state. You can click on your state on the map to get details and contact information on Medicare specific to your state.

Medicare Forms and Other

Assistance

All necessary forms for Medicare are located on the <u>Medicare.gov form page</u>. Most of the forms are identified by their purpose. For example, one form is linked from the phrase "I want to file a claim for services and/or supplies that I got (Patient Request for Medical Payment form/CMS-149S)." This simplifies the process of finding the right form for what you need.

If you have questions, use one of the boxes on the right side of the screen to look for more information or to contact someone who can help.

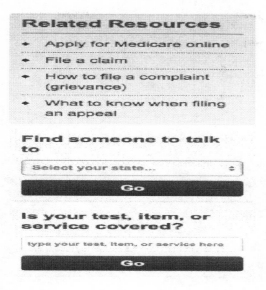

There is also a <u>publication page</u> that you can take some time to review to stay current on the latest news, research, laws, and details about Medicare.

| Find health & drug plans |
| Find & compare doctors, hospitals, & other providers |
| Get help paying costs |
| Find suppliers of medical equipment & supplies |
| **Medicare forms** |
| Publications |
| Medicare & You |

You can also access forms from the CMS site. While it is not quite as easy to find what you need, there are a lot more forms here. The sites are related, so between the two sites, you should be able to find all of the forms you need.

If you have trouble navigating the site, you can check out cahaba.com. While you should not start your search for forms here, it does contain all of the forms you need and is organized differently than the government sites. If you feel that you need some additional help you can probably find what you need on this site. However, keep in mind that it is a commercial site and some of the details may not be as straightforward as it is on the government sites.

You can also go to Google.com and enter the name of your state and its Medicare forms to get any information that may be required for your state. Because states have a certain amount of control, Medicare may vary from state to state. Make sure you have not missed any information you may need or forms specific to your state. Keep in mind that some states provide more assistance than others. If you don't find what you need on your state site, check with one of the two federal government sites for more information. You should not be trying to get information from friends and family in other states – and always take what they say with a grain of salt.

Appendix B –Tips

Although many people are eligible for Medicare, many do not take full advantage of the different Parts and supplemental coverage. To help you ensure you are getting the most out of your Medicare coverage, this appendix provides tips and information that will help you get started finding out what the best options are for your specific needs.

Get Started Researching Before Your 65th Birthday

There are so many different plans and options that it can be a bit overwhelming.

The best way to ensure you have the right coverage for Medicare is to start doing your research well in advance of your 65th birthday.

It should be part of your retirement planning because most Medicare Parts have associated costs – so it should be part of your retirement planning – long before you are eligible for Medicare.

If you are nearing your 65th birthday (or if it has already past), you need to set aside the time to really examine your options. It is possible that you will need to pay a late enrollment fee, but it will be best to have the coverage you need before you need it. Even if you have Medicare, you are going to need to pay for it. The longer you wait, the more you are likely to pay per month, and the harder it will be to budget for it since you did not plan for healthcare coverage before retiring. This can be true even if you continue to work after you retire because you will have complications in your taxes.

For those who need further assistance, there are things like Extra Help (covered under

Payment Programs near the end of Appendix B) that can reduce the cost of insurance. It is best to get the medical attention you need, especially as you age. The longer you procrastinate, the more severe the problems will be (and it is likely you will have more problems than just the original medical issue) and the more costly it will be.

You can begin the enrollment process three months before you turn 65. Doing so ensures that you have medical coverage should anything happen on or right after your 65th birthday. It also lets you sit back and enjoy your birthday. For those who retire on their 65th birthday, it really makes it easier to enjoy your retirement right from the beginning.

REVIEW ALL OF YOUR OPTIONS

There are so many different options. Medicare is a lot like a mix and match where you can take a little bit of many different things or you can switch plans to something that better meets your needs. Healthcare changes every year, making it a great idea to look into all of your options every year. Because there are so many options, you really need to ensure that you go through all of them the first time you enroll. Keep all of your comparisons so that you can more quickly go through your options next year.

Put it on your calendar to do an analysis on your options every year around the end of September to the beginning of November. That will mean that you have the information you need when the enrollment period begins. You can ask any questions you have about the options and plans and enroll early so that you don't have to worry about procrastinating past the deadline – or missing a better plan because you had to rush through the enrollment period.

Making Medicare planning part of your annual fall activities will be similar to paying taxes, but with the benefit of possibly getting better coverage or minimizing your budget increases every year. When you are living on a fixed income, the more you can do to keep your healthcare costs down the better.

COMPARE YOUR MEDICARE COSTS TO YOUR RETIREMENT BUDGET

One of the biggest mistakes people make is to neglect Medicare in their retirement planning. Too often, people think about their retirement savings, investments, and lifestyle changes, but they completely neglect to consider Medicare or healthcare coverage costs. If you are nearly retirement age, you really need to get a better understanding of Medicare to ensure that you do not miss out on the best options for your specific situation. If you are nearing retirement and Medicare eligibility, it is going to be very difficult to make time to understand what you need to know about Medicare to make a well-informed decision. And thinking that you can fix it later will likely mean you end up either paying more or you miss out on something you need, and will result in a late payment or a large medical bill later.

To properly budget for Medicare, you must take the time to understand the different parts and the premiums that apply to each. Your Part B premium is not going to cover prescriptions you need, and trying to get Part D later will mean an additional charge if you did not enroll for this part when you enroll in Parts A and B.

The likelihood that you will have more health concerns at 65 and older is great, so it really needs to be something you consider as part of your retirement plan. It is really too late to start shopping once you have a medical emergency after you turn 65.

BE CAUTIOUS OF MEDICARE FRAUD

Medicare is a highly regulated benefit, one that scammers and con artists try to use to their advantage because most people do not understand their rights. While removing your Social Security Number from your card and using a new Medicare Number will help prevent some types of fraud, there are other ways people can use your Medicare benefits without you benefiting.

MEDICARE MAY NOT BE YOUR BEST

OPTION

While every American over 65 is eligible for Medicare, it is not always the best option. Some companies and agencies offer much better coverage after retirement that can save you a considerable sum. It can't hurt to inquire at the HR department to see if they have insurance for retirees. If they do, take that into account when considering healthcare coverage after retirement. If it is better coverage at roughly the same cost as Medicare, you won't need to pay for inferior coverage.

Take the Time to Get Screened for Payment Programs

Living on a fixed income can really change a person's perspective, and suddenly being responsible for paying premiums after being enrolled in automatic payments from work can shed light on something most people don't consider. Seeing just how much insurance costs every month can make it difficult to meet a fixed budget every month.

The best way to manage these kinds of issues is to look into programs that have been set up to help those on Medicare. Though it can really help, Medicare can be difficult for some people to afford once they are retired.

Start by going to the Medicare interactive page that will walk you through a number of options and help you determine your eligibility for some of those programs.

• Extra Help is designed specifically to help those who have Medicare Part D. Even with help from Medicare to reduce prescription costs, life-saving drugs can be a burden on a fixed income. This program is designed to help ensure people who require medication are able to afford that medication if they are on Medicare.

• If you aren't eligible for Medicare, typically because you are younger than 65 years old, you may qualify for Medicaid. It is a separate program that provides assistance for those who cannot afford healthcare coverage on their own. It can provide assistance for prescription drugs as well.

• State programs are something you will need to research based on the state in which you live, but many states do have financial assistance for lower income families and seniors. One such program is the state pharmaceutical assistance program. Not all states participate in this program, but enough do that it will be well worth your time to see if your state does. It can provide assistance in paying for prescription medications.

• Some pharmacies that are part of government-funded hospitals also provide additional medical assistance to lower income families and seniors. As long as you are enrolled in Medicare, they can help reduce your costs. Find out if any of the hospitals or clinics near you offer this kind of assistance.

REVIEW LOCAL PHYSICIANS AND PHARMACIES

Not all offices and pharmacies participate in Medicare, so your new Medicare coverage will not cover the costs you incur when you visit them. It is important that you make sure your trusted physicians, specialists, hospital, and pharmacy will take your Medicare when the time comes. It is best to know now so before you incur costs that end up coming out of your pocket.

Recommendations:

Roxanne Robertson is a licensed professional insurance agent, who represents over 20 of the top A rated insurance carriers. Licensed in over 40 states, she is able to help most Americans select the best option for their specific needs, as well as complete the enrollment process. Please don't hesitate to contact her with any questions.

Business Number: 913-593-1291

(Mon-Fri) 9:00 A.M. - 6:00 P.M Central Standard

(Sat) 10:00 AM - 2:00 P.M. Central Standard

or

Roxanne@Medigapselect.com

ABOUT THE AUTHOR

Mario Robertson is a Marine Corps Veteran, who studied Health Care Management at Park University. Upon completion of his bachelor's degree he produces non-fiction informational books, as well as volunteers his services at the local VA. Mario is also a licensed insurance agent who serviced over 35 states during his time as a broker. He currently resides with his wife, and 2 children in the great state of Kansas.

OTHER BOOKS BY (MARIO ROBERTSON)

AirBnB: A Beginning Users Guide

Inner Peace: The inconvenient Truth

Thanks for Reading!

I hope you enjoyed reading Medicare 2018 - 2020 The Complete Comprehensive Guide

Make sure you get a copy of the books mentioned above.

If you learned anything new, or found this book useful, please take one minute to leave an honest review on Amazon.